LIPOSUCTION: YES OR NO?

AUTHOR:
Bilikis O. Yakubu

3

Table of Contents

What is Liposuction?

Liposuction, also called lipoplasty, liposculpture, lipectomy, or lipo, is a type of cosmetic surgery that breaks up and "sucks" fat from the body. It is a procedure that removes fat that you can't seem to get rid of through diet and exercise. Just like any other surgical procedure, liposuction comes with both medical and aesthetic risks that patients should be made aware of prior to undergoing the operation. Liposuction is however fairly routine for experienced plastic surgeons and when performed by talented professionals, patients are mostly satisfied with the outcome.

It is often used on the abdomen, thighs, buttocks, neck, chin, upper and backs of the arms, calves, and back.

A plastic or dermatologic surgeon usually does the procedure on your hips, belly, thighs, buttocks, back, arms, and under the chin or face to improve their shape. But liposuction can also be done with other plastic surgeries, including facelifts, breast reductions, and tummy tucks. The fat is removed through a hollow instrument, known as a cannula. This is inserted under the skin. A powerful, high-pressure vacuum is applied to the cannula.

Liposuction is the most common cosmetic operation in the United States. More than 300,000 procedures are carried out in the United States each year with costs ranging from roughly $2,000-3,500.

People who undergo liposuction usually have a stable body weight but would like to remove undesirable deposits of body fat in specific parts of the body.

Liposuction is not an overall weight-loss method. It is not a treatment for obesity.

The procedure does not remove cellulite, dimples, or stretch marks. The aim is esthetic. It suits those who wish to change and enhance the contour of their body.

Liposuction permanently removes fat cells, altering the shape of the body. However, if the patient does not lead a healthy lifestyle after the operation, there is a risk that the remaining fat cells will grow bigger.

The amount of fat that can be safely removed is limited.

There are some risks, including infection, numbness, and scarring. If too much fat is removed, there may be lumpiness or dents in the skin. The surgical risks appear to be linked to the amount of fat removed.

Types and Benefits

Types of Liposuction

There are just a few different liposuction techniques. But what they all have in common is the use of a thin tube, called a cannula, connected to a vacuum to suction the fat from your body.

- Tumescent **liposuction** is the most common technique. Your surgeon injects a sterile solution into the area where the fat is to be removed. It consists of saline --

which is salt water - along with lidocaine and epinephrine. The solution makes it easier to suction the fat with less blood loss and pain.

- **Ultrasound-assisted liposuction,** or UAL, uses sound wave energy under your skin to rupture the cell walls of the fat. This liquefies the fat so it can be suctioned out.

- **Laser-assisted liposuction,** or SmartLipo, uses a laser to produce a burst of energy to liquefy the fat.

Benefits

Liposuction is normally done for cosmetic purposes, but it is sometimes used to treat certain conditions.

These include:

Lymphedema: A chronic, or long-term, condition in which excess fluid known as lymph collects in tissues, causing edema, or swelling. The edema commonly occurs in the arms or legs. Liposuction is sometimes used to reduce swelling, discomfort, and pain.

Gynecomastia: Sometimes fat accumulates under a man's breasts.

Lipodystrophy syndrome: Fat accumulates in one part of the body and is lost in another. Liposuction can improve the patient's appearance by providing a more natural looking body fat distribution.

Extreme weight loss after obesity: A person with morbid obesity who loses at least 40 percent of their BMI may need treatment to remove excess skin and other abnormalities.

Lipomas: These are benign, fatty tumors.

Risks

Liposuction, like other cosmetic procedures, will have both medical and aesthetic risks. Medical risks are those which can be compromising to your health, while aesthetic risks are those which alter the way you look without harming your overall health.

Medical Risks:

Seroma

Seroma is a build up of fluid which can occur after liposuction. A common reason for this to happen is damage to the lymphatics caused by the cannula, which is the instrument used to remove the fat. Smaller seromas can be absorbed back into the body naturally but larger ones have the potential to become infected requiring medical attention.

Anesthesia Reaction

Liposuction requires you go under general anesthesia which can vary in length of time depending on the area treated. Anesthesia always poses mild to severe risks. During your consultation, your surgeon will determine whether you are a good candidate for general anesthesia to avoid any major risks.

Lidocaine Reaction

Lidocaine is the most commonly used drug in liposuction, it reduces pain by blocking the signal from nerve endings to the brain. Although lidocaine is safe for most people, it may cause adverse side effects in some. If you have experienced any reaction to lidocaine in the past it is critical that you discuss this with your doctor.

Infection

While not common, infection is always a risk with liposuction. Too much movement or pressure on the area too soon after surgery can be the leading risk factor in becoming infected. To avoid this from happening, it is crucial that the patient follows post-surgical care guidelines.

Fat Embolism

Fat Embolism is when fat becomes trapped in the blood vessel and travels through the bloodstream to major organs. Fat embolism occurs when fat that has been broken up is carried to another part of the body by the blood stream. This is one of the more dangerous risks of liposuction and requires urgent medical attention.

Internal Puncture

Though extremely rare, it is possible for a cannula to puncture an internal organ by getting too close to it during the removal of fat. This requires urgent care.

Aesthetic Risks:

Scarring

Because your subcutaneous layer is being penetrated during the procedure, some scarring will be inevitable; however, a skilled surgeon will use techniques that conceal scarring in less visible places. Your doctor will also suggest a post-surgical care routine designed to minimize scarring.

Ask about topical creams to help reduce any scarring. Also protect any scars from exposure to the sun. With appropriate care and time, they fade into minor blemishes.

Loose Skin

Loose skin may occur after liposuction as a result of the fat removal. Older patients and patients with less skin elasticity are at the highest risk of having loose skin after the procedure. There are however ways this can be treated including additional surgery or even by toning the muscles underneath.

Irregular Contouring

An uneven distribution of subcutaneous fat pockets is a common complication in liposuction. To mitigate the risk, it's important to find an experienced and highly-qualified surgeon who will be able to create the most flattering contours possible.

Also, don't forget to wear liposuction compression garments for better results.

Liposuction is a serious surgery with multiple risks. It's important to discuss all the risks of liposuction with your doctor before having the procedure.

- **Risks during surgery**

- The risks during surgery include:

- puncture wounds or injuries to other organs

- anesthesia complications

- burns from equipment, such as ultrasound probes

- nerve damage

- shock

- death

Risks immediately after the procedure

The risks after the procedure include:

- blood clot in the lungs

- too much fluid in the lungs

- fat clots

- infections

- hematoma (bleeding under the skin)

- seroma (fluid leaking under the skin)

- edema (swelling)

- skin necrosis (the death of skin cells)

- reactions to anesthesia and other medications

- heart and kidney problems

- death

Risks during recovery

The risks during recovery include:

- problems with the shape or contours of the body

- wavy, dimpled, or bumpy skin

- numbness, bruising, pain, swelling, and soreness

- infections

- fluid imbalances

- scars

- changes in skin sensation and feeling

- skin color changes

- problems with healing

What are the long-term side effects of liposuction?

The long-term side effects of liposuction can vary. Liposuction permanently removes fat cells from the targeted areas of the body. So, if you gain weight, the fat will still be stored in different parts of the body. The new fat can appear deeper under the skin, and it can be dangerous if it grows around the liver or heart.

Some people experience permanent nerve damage and changes to skin sensation. Others may develop depressions or indentations in the areas that were suctioned, or may have bumpy or wavy skin that doesn't go away.

Weighing the Risk and Reward

Like with any invasive surgery, liposuction comes with its own set of risks and risk level which varies from patient to patient. Liposuction is generally safe especially when performed by a highly skilled surgeon in a facility that meets all healthy and safety standards.

When it comes to surgery, understanding the risks and trusting a skilled surgeon is your best defence against complications. There are always risks when going under the knife, but with careful planning and close attention to detail, you can minimize a lot of those risks. A patient's best protection during surgery is someone in their corner — who will be there for them before, during and after an operation.

The operation

Before the operation, patients will need to undergo some health tests to ensure they are fit for surgery.

The following recommendations may be made.

People who use regular aspirin and anti-inflammatory drugs should stop taking them at least 2 weeks before surgery.

Women may be asked to stop taking the contraceptive pill.

Patients with anemia may be asked to take iron supplements. The individual will need to sign a consent form. This confirms that they are fully aware of the risks, benefits, and possible alternatives to the procedure

What to expect with liposuction

Liposuction requires going under anesthesia for the procedure. This means you won't feel any pain during the liposuction surgery. However, you'll feel pain after the procedure. Recovery can also be painful.

Depending on the area of the body that is being treated, liposuction can have different effects and recovery times. Some procedures are performed in an outpatient center, while others require a hospital stay.

Liposuction is performed under general anesthesia. A highly qualified anesthesiologist will determine the proper dosing to safely provide that will keep you unconscious for the duration of the surgery.

After coming out of the anesthesia you will likely be in pain as well as feel pain and/or general discomfort during the recovery phase. All of this is a completely normal part of the process and nothing to be concerned about. Your doctor will be able to discuss treatments to make your post-surgery pain more manageable. It's common to experience swelling, pain, bruising, numbness and soreness after liposuction.

To minimize pain before the procedure, you can:

talk to your doctor about pain concerns

discuss the type of anesthesia that will be used

ask about any medications you can take before the procedure

To minimize pain after the procedure:

take all prescribed medications,
including **pain pills**

wear the recommended compression
garments

keep the drains after surgery in
place based on your doctor's
recommendations

rest and try to relax

drink fluids

avoid salt, which can increase
swelling (edema)

Am I a Good Candidate?

You'll want to have realistic expectations. Liposuction won't get rid of cellulite, so if you hoped you'd come out of surgery without any, you're out of luck.

Liposuction is a surgical procedure, and with it comes risks. So you need to be in good health before you get it. Doctors don't recommend the procedure if you have health problems with blood flow or have heart disease, diabetes, or a weak immune system.

Some people are good candidates for liposuction, and others should avoid it. Talk to your doctor to determine if liposuction is the right option for you. Discuss your concerns with them.

Good candidates for **lipos**uction include people who:

- don't have a lot of excess skin

- have good skin elasticity

- have good muscle tone

- Be within 30% of your ideal weight

- Have firm, elastic skin

- have fat deposits that won't go away with diet or exercise

- are in good physical shape and overall health

- aren't overweight or obese

- don't smoke

You should avoid liposuction if you:

- smoke

- have chronic health problems

- have a weak immune system

- are overweight

- have saggy skin

- have a history of diabetes, cardiovascular

disease, deep vein thrombosis (DVT), or seizures

- take medications that can increase the risk of bleeding, such as blood thinners